Vatsyayana

Love

THE *KAMA SUTRA* GUIDE TO THE
MANAGEMENT OF MEN

➤►◄◄

P
PROFILE BOOKS

First published in Great Britain in 2001 by
Profile Books Ltd
58A Hatton Garden
London EC1N 8LX
www.profilebooks.co.uk

Introduction and text selection copyright
© Jeremy Scott 2001

Text extracts selected from the *Kama Sutra*; translated by Sir
Richard Burton and F. F. Arbuthnot; privately printed in
London and Benares in 1883.

A CIP catalogue record for this book is available from the
British Library.

ISBN 1 86197 358 6

Cover design by the Senate
Cover and frontispiece illustration by Clifford Harper
Text design by Geoff Green
Typeset in Van Dijck by MacGuru
info@macguru.org.uk

Printed and bound in Great Britain by
Bookmarque Ltd, Croydon, Surrey

Contents

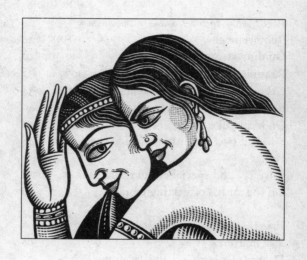

The *Kama Sutra* is a title familiar everywhere. It is one of the most famous and least read books in the world; almost everyone knows about it and most believe – mistakenly – that they know what it contains.

But the book is much wider in scope than the sexual treatise many imagine it to be. It is nothing less than a lifestyle manual for sophisticated city-living men and women who want to extract the most from life. Then as now.

About its author, Vatsyayana, little is known beyond the fact that he was a Brahman, or member of the highest caste in the Hindu caste system, living in the cities of Pataliputra and Benares in India during the fourth century AD; and that he composed his celebrated work 'for the benefit of mankind while following the life of a religious student and wholly engaged in the contemplation of the Deity'.

The *Kama Sutra*, with its acute psychological insight and detailed knowledge of the emotional and physical characteristics of women and men, is clearly not the work of a writer who is young. Almost the only thing that can be said with certainty about the author is that he was a very mature student indeed. His book is the result not just of observation and study but of personal experience, as he admits himself.

That he should have written his erotic manual while studying religion and 'wholly engaged in the contemplation of the Deity' sounds somewhat incongruous to a Westerner, but Hindus had an entirely different attitude to sex. Sexual guilt found no place in their lives or religion; for them there was nothing smutty or obscene about sex. On the contrary, it had a divine significance and was held in reverence as an almost sacramental act.

According to Hindu mythology, the world came into being through energy (*prakriti*) acting upon matter (*purusha*). This was symbolised by the union of the god Shiva with Shakti, whose respective signs are the *lingam* and *yoni*, the penis and vagina. Sex was to be celebrated as a holy act of creation.

The aim of life was salvation, in the form of liberation from the world and from the repetitive cycle of reincarnation. And one of the intermediate ways of achieving that liberation was in fully realised and mutually satisfying sex with a partner of the opposite gender. Physically and emotionally, one merges into the other; their duality melts away in the act so that they become one.

Vatsyayana's and the Hindu view was that women and men should above all else seek harmony in the way they conduct their lives. To achieve this state of stability and calm they should balance three activities, *Dharma*, *Artha* and *Kama*, in such a way that they do not conflict or destabilise one another. None of these activities should be neglected, nor should one be pursued at the expense of the other two.

Dharma is the due observance of a moral code. This is learnt from Holy Writ and religious teachers and leads to *Moksha*, liberation from the necessity of reincarnation.

Artha is work, business and politics, the pursuit of a job, and acquiring of position and wealth. It should be learned, Vatsyayana says, 'from king's officers and merchants well versed in the ways of commerce'.

Kama is the enjoyment of the five senses: hearing, feeling, seeing, tasting and smelling, assisted by the mind together with the soul.

'The ingredient of this is a peculiar contact between the organ of sense and its object, and the consciousness of pleasure which arises from that contact.' *Kama* is to be learnt from the *Kama Sutra* and 'from the practice of citizens'.

About the practice of citizens in India in the fourth century BC (the period about which Vatsyayana is writing, when in the West the civilisation of ancient Greece was at its height and both Socrates and Plato were alive) a certain amount is known. Poetry, prose epics, paintings, and most explicitly temple carvings portraying women and men serenely engaged in an all-embracing range of sexual activities suggest that it was in many ways a highly sophisticated culture.

Vatsyayana's book is directed at a city readership, a prosperous, leisured middle class with time and money on its hands and an instinct for pleasure. The first section of the *Kama Sutra* reproduced in this volume is addressed to women only, the second to men.

The sort of man Vatsyayana is writing for is a *Nagaraka*, a member of a self-declared elite. The *Nagaraka* may be a noble, a government official, a warrior, a merchant or someone who has made it out of nowhere from sheer ability. He may or may not work, has a high disposable income and lives either in his own or a rented house in a fashionable area of town, looked after by servants. Educated and cultured, he is not wholly devoted to pleasure, but also follows intellectual and artistic pursuits. He keeps himself fit through sport and hunting.

Vatsyayana goes into considerable detail describing the sort of house a *Nagaraka* should live in. It should have a very impressive entrance hall. Between this hall and the private apartments, which no guests are allowed to enter, lies the antechamber, which must be vast. In the centre of this room stands a wide divan covered with white cloth. This is where the *Nagaraka* usually sits himself, and where he seats the business associates, scholars and friends who visit in the course of every day. Not far from this divan is another, equally large. At the head of this bed is a large mirror, and on the floor beside it a rug spread with bolsters and cushions. Shelves contain dice, games, books, flower necklaces, ointments, pots of scent and jars of betel leaves. A spittoon stands conveniently placed. Music is provided by caged birds in the courtyard outside the window.

The *Nagaraka*'s lifestyle and personal grooming regimen is described. He has a bath daily, a massage every other day and uses soap twice a week. Every fourth day he has his beard and moustache trimmed; every fifth day his pubic and under-arm hair is shaved. Additionally, Vatsyayana says, 'he should always scent himself to disguise the smell of sweat and be pleasant to contact'.

Much of the *Nagaraka*'s morning is spent in his bathroom and dressing room where, assisted by hairdresser and servants, he is prepared for his day. After lunch he meets his manager, lawyer and secretary to deal with business matters. Then, Vatsyayana says, he should do something relaxing such as teaching a parrot to speak, before taking a well-earned siesta.

Refreshed, he rises from his rest to change and put on his jewels in preparation for the evening ahead. Later, 'having listened to music, he returns with some friends to his dwelling where, with wine and incense, he awaits the arrival of the women invited for the night . . .'.

Such was Vatsyayana's male readership, whose equivalent today is probably reading GQ magazine along with the 'Style' and 'Culture' sections of the *Sunday Times*. But the first part of this edition of his book is addressed not to men but to women, and specifically to *Ganikas*.

The *Ganika* is not the *Nagaraka*'s female equivalent, but his counterpart. She is a woman of intelligence and culture, sophistication and style. Always perfectly groomed, she is socially highly skilled and duly respected and esteemed. Often the companion of a king or minister, the *Ganika* is to be found at the best houses, the most fashionable parties and also at more intimate occasions.

And, always and everywhere, it is she who is in charge of the game . . .

Origins of the Kama Sutra
Vatsyayana ascribes the origins of his book to a mythological work in 1000 chapters by Nandi, female companion of Shiva. Supposedly condensed into 500 chapters in the eighth century

BC, during the centuries which followed, this text was reworked many times by sages and teachers, who added commentaries updating and expanding it. The book multiplied from one volume into many, as commentaries and original text became inseparable. Vatsyayana's work is not original, but a compilation and part of a long tradition.

The translation

In the 1870s this unwieldy mass of material, written in Sanskrit and dispersed all over India, was collected by two men, who embarked on the awesome task of translating it into English.

F. F. Arbuthnot was an expert in Sanskrit, a quiet, unassertive Indian civil servant who did not get married until retirement. Sir Richard Burton was one of the most extraordinary men of his century. Army officer, explorer, anthropologist, expert swordsman, scholar, writer, he spoke twenty-five languages with a further fifteen dialects. He was also bi-sexual and was described as having 'sex in the head'.

Burton's interest was academic, but also personal. Officers in the Indian Army invariably employed a *bubu*, a girl who provided sexual services and also worked in the house. But as Burton was the only officer in his regiment even halfway competent in the local language he was the only one to understand what the *bubus* thought of these officers, including himself. Indian males had been trained from an early age to please, and to delay orgasm for thirty minutes and longer. But these gorgeously dressed young Englishmen reached their climax within seconds. The *bubus* laughed at their strutting self-regard and incompetence, calling them cockerels.

The humiliation of this lesson stayed with Burton, as did his fascination with performance and sexual detail. While leading an expedition in search of the source of the Nile, he measured a particularly impressive local penis, both resting and erect. (It was, he recorded, significantly larger than the standard African norm of six to seven inches, while the European averaged six inches and the Arab five.) He noted that African males made better lovers; they were so laid-back they took much longer to come than excitable Arabs.

As an anthropologist, Burton believed the key to understanding any society lies in how it regards and treats women. But his earliest studies were on males. As a young subaltern he was asked by his commanding officer to investigate Karachi's thriving gay brothels, where many of the garrison's soldiers passed their off-duty hours. Disguised as a Persian merchant, Burton did so. His report covers every variety of pederasty, fellatio, transvestism, infibulation, troilism and group sex, and includes the detail that young intact boys received twice the price of eunuchs as 'the scrotum of the unmutilated boy can be used as a kind of bridle for directing the movements of the animal'.

To describe Burton only in this way, however, is misleading, diminishing and grossly unfair to him. He was intrepid, erudite, outspoken, had a will of steel, didn't give a damn for authority and possessed a brilliance of mind which at times touched genius. He was a man of many, often conflicting, parts – including the character of a sexual obsessive.

Unknown to the West, the *Kama Sutra* had existed in some form as a socio-sexual manual for 3000 years. In Burton it met its ideal translator; book and man are in perfect harmony.

Burton and Arbuthnot's work was unpublishable in their own time for reasons of obscenity. In 1883 the two men printed a limited edition 'for private subscribers only'. The book was published in England for the first time only in 1963.

Vatsyayana introduces himself and explains his work

-➤-><-◄-

After reading and considering the works of ancient authors and thinking over the meaning of the rules given by them, the *Kama Sutra* was composed, according to the precepts of Holy Writ for the benefit of the world, by myself, while leading the life of a religious student and wholly engaged in the contemplation of the Deity.

This work is not intended to be used merely as an instrument for satisfying our desires. A person acquainted with the true principles of this science of love, who preserves their Dharma, Artha, and Kama, and has regard for the practices of the other people, is sure to obtain mastery over their senses.

In short, an intelligent and prudent person, without becoming a slave to their passions, will obtain success in everything they may undertake.

PART I
How to select, manage and make use of men

◆━◆

Some learned men object to women studying the *Kama Sutra*, saying they should not be allowed to do so.

But personally this author believes this objection is without value, for women already *know* the science of love. Yet it is certain that in this science, as in many others, although the science may be familiar to all, very few persons are acquainted with the rules and laws on which the science is based.

Experience shows us that some women, such as the daughters of princes and their ministers, and society women, are in fact well versed in the *Kama Sutra*. Others, even young maids, should study it . . .

Necessary psycho-sexual arts

A woman of good disposition and beauty, versed in these arts, obtains the name of a *Ganika*, or woman of high quality, and receives a seat of honour in an assembly of men. Respected by the king, praised by learned men, her favour is sought by all and she becomes an object of universal regard.

Even if such a woman becomes separated from her partner, and falls into distress, she can support herself easily, even in a foreign country, by means of these arts. Even the bare knowledge of them gives her attractiveness, though the practice of them may only be possible or otherwise according to the circumstances of each case . . .

Intuitive skill

At all times and in all places there has ever been a little rivalry between the chaste and the unchaste. But while some women are born with such knowledge and follow the instincts of their nature in every class of society, it has been truly said by some authors that every woman has got an inkling of those skills in her nature and knows how to make herself desirable.

The subtlety of women, their wonderful perceptiveness, their knowledge, and their intuitive understanding of men and all things are shown in the following pages.

Requirements

✦✦✦

A woman should have the following characteristics:

She should be possessed of beauty and an amiable nature, with a liking for good qualities in other people and also a liking for wealth. She should take delight in sexual unions resulting from love, be of firm mind, and in the same class as the man with regard to sexual enjoyment.

She should always desire to acquire experience and knowledge, and have a liking for social gatherings and for the arts.

She should possess intelligence and good manners, be straightforward in behaviour, and show gratitude; consider well the future before she acts; be sophisticated and socially aware; converse without loud laughter, coarseness, anger, dullness or stupidity; have knowledge of the *Kama Sutra*, and be skilled in all the arts of love.

Guiding strategy

❯❯❮❮

By having intercourse with men *Ganikas* obtain sexual pleasure, as well as their own maintenance.

Now when a woman takes up with a man from love the action is natural, but when she does so for the purpose of getting money her action is artificial. In the latter case, however, she should conduct herself as if her love were indeed natural, because men place their confidence in those women who apparently love them.

In making known her love for a man a *Ganika* should give the appearance of being wholly without greed, and for the sake of her future advantage she should abstain from acquiring money from him by unlawful means.

Staging and motive

Elegantly attired wearing her jewels and ornaments, a woman should position herself in such places where she will be observed and noticed by men. But if she shows herself off shamelessly it will diminish her value.

She should form friendships with such people as will enable her to separate men from other women, and attach them to herself.

The reasons for doing so are to acquire wealth, to repair her misfortunes, and to protect herself from being bullied by persons with whom she may have dealings of some kind, such as the police, court officials, powerful men, parasites, hairdressers and beggars.

Marks

The following kinds of men may be taken up with for the purpose of getting money:

Men possessed of unfailing sources of income.
Young men.
Men who consider themselves handsome.
Men holding places of authority.
Men who have secured their means of livelihood without difficulty.
Men who are always praising themselves.
One who is a eunuch but wishes to be thought a man.
One who has influence with the king or his ministers.
One who is always fortunate.
An ascetic who is internally troubled with desire.
An only son whose father is wealthy.

A better class of john

On the other hand there is another sort of man who is to be resorted to for reasons of love and fame. Such men are as follows:

Men of high birth, learned and experienced in the world.

Energetic and eloquent men, skilled in various arts.

Intelligent men possessed of great minds, far-seeing into the future.

Liberal men free from anger, who are affectionate and sociable.

Men of perfect physique, strong, not addicted to drink, and of sexual prowess.

Rich men, free from anger and suspicion, who like women.

Discards

The following kinds of men are not fit to be taken up:

One who is consumptive, sickly, whose mouth contains worms or whose breath smells of excrement.
One whose wife is dear to him.
One who is suspicious, avaricious, pitiless, or a thief.
One who does not care for respect or disrespect.
One who can be gained over even by his enemies by means of money.
One who is extremely bashful.

Reasons for a man

——>>—<<——

Ancient writers are of the opinion that the reasons for a woman acquiring a man are love, fear, money, celebrity, pleasure, pity, sorrow, constant sexual intercourse, the desire for a friend, shame, his similarity to someone else, convenience, the search for good luck and poverty.

But this author believes that the desire of wealth, freedom from misfortune, and love are the only reasons.

Choosing a lover: the guiding rules

→>←←

Most authorities state that, when a *Ganika* has the chance of an equal gain from two lovers, preference should be given to the one who is prepared to give her the things she wants.

But this author believes that she should choose the one who gives money. Money cannot be taken back like some other things, and it is the means of procuring anything that may be wished for.

Of such gifts as jewellery, perfume, clothes, furniture, fittings and money, money is to be preferred. It is superior to all the others.

Rich or useful?

When there are two lovers, one of whom is generous and the other ready to perform some service, there is an opinion that the first is to be preferred.

But this author holds the opinion that a man who has performed a service thinks he has gained his object when he has done something once, but a generous man does not consider what he has given before.

The woman's choice must be guided by her estimate of the future benefit she is likely to gain by taking up with either of them.

Grateful . . . or generous?

When one of the two lovers is grateful and the other generous, some sages say the generous one is to be preferred.

But this author believes the former should be chosen because generous men are often haughty, plain-spoken, and lack consideration toward others. Even though these generous men have been on friendly terms for a long time, yet if they see any fault in the *Ganika*, or are told lies about her by some other women, they do not care for past services but leave abruptly. On the other hand the grateful man does not at once break off from her on account of his regard for the trouble she has taken to please him.

But in this case also the choice is to be guided with respect to what may happen in future.

Money . . . or help in avoiding a disaster?

When the chance of getting money and the chance of avoiding some disaster come at the same time, the sages are of the opinion that the chance of getting money should be preferred.

But this author holds that money has only a limited importance, while a disaster that is once averted may never occur again.

Here, however, the choice should be guided by the greatness or smallness of the disaster.

As a guiding principle

In considering her present gains and her future welfare, a *Ganika* should avoid such persons who have gained their wealth with very great difficulty, and also avoid those who have become selfish and hard-hearted through their success in becoming the favourites of kings.

Remember . . . denial

only stimulates

➤><◄

A *Ganika* should not sacrifice money to love, because money is the chief thing to be attended to. But in cases of fear etc, she should pay attention to power, position, and other qualities a man may possess.

Most importantly, though she may be invited, she should not at once consent to sexual union, for men are apt to despise things which are easily acquired.

On living like a wife . . .

✦✦✦

When a *Ganika* has many suitors, she should not confine herself to a single lover if she is able to obtain a price from all of them.

If, however, she can obtain great gain from a single lover she may resort to him alone and live with him like a wife.

Don't love . . . but seem to love

When a *Ganika* is living as a wife with her lover she should behave like a chaste woman and do everything to his satisfaction.

Her aim should be to give him pleasure, but she should not become attached to him though behaving as if she were really attached.

Peace and prosperity

A woman who chooses to lead in this
manner the life of a wife is not troubled by
too many lovers, and yet obtains great
abundance of wealth.

Inspiring love

A woman should do the following things to cause the man to love her:

Treasuring his flowers and gifts as tokens of affection; asking for the mixture of betel nut and leaves that has remained uneaten by him; expressing wonder at his knowledge and skill in sexual intercourse; continually practising the ways of enjoyment taught by him, and according to his liking; keeping his secrets; telling him her own desires and secrets; concealing her anger; looking at him with apparent anxiety when he is wrapped in thought; showing a liking for that which he likes; being in high or low spirits according to the state he is in himself; expressing a curiosity to meet his family; remaining silent when he is asleep, intoxicated, or sick; being very attentive when he describes his good actions, and reciting them afterwards to his praise;

abstaining from putting on her ornaments or eating food when he is in pain, sick, or low-spirited; listening to all his stories, except those that relate to her rivals; expressing sorrow if he falls down; wearing anything he may have given her; wishing to accompany him if he is banished from the country by the king; expressing a desire not to live after him; putting on ornaments every day; not acting too freely with him; placing his hand on her loins; looking on her own wealth and his without distinction; abstaining from going to public assemblies without him; accompanying him when he desires to do so; taking delight in using things previously used by him and in eating food he has left uneaten; adapting her tastes, dispositions and actions to his liking; venerating his family, his disposition, his skill, his learning, his culture, his complexion, his friends, his qualities, his age, and his sweet temper; and lastly abstaining from sorcery.

Such is the guidance for a Ganika living like a wife. To conclude, there are two verses on the subject . . .

→>-<←

The extent of the love of women is not known, even to those who are the objects of their affection, on account of the subtlety, the avarice, and natural intelligence of womankind.

Women are hardly ever known in their true light, though they may love men, or become indifferent towards them, may give them delight, or abandon them, or may extract from them all the wealth that they may possess.

Policy

>+>+<+

Even at some cost to herself a *Ganika* should make every effort to get to know and to cultivate prosperous and successful people, and also those it is dangerous to avoid or slight in any way.

Whatever the difficulties, she must become acquainted with wealthy and liberal men who, when pleased, will give her a large sum of money even for very little.

Price . . . and special
circumstances

→>—<←

There are some situations where a *Ganika* may choose to take only a token fee from the man.

These are the following:

When she wishes to keep some particular man from some other woman; or wishes to get him away from some woman to whom he may be attached; or to deprive some woman from the gains she is making from him; or if the *Ganika* thinks she would improve her status, or become desirable to all men by uniting herself with this particular lover; or if she requires his help in averting some misfortune; or is really attached to him and loves him; or needs his assistance in order to injure somebody; or wishes to repay a favour; or wants to enjoy sex with him merely from lustful desire . . . for any of the above reasons she should agree to take from him only a small sum of money in a friendly way.

Promise

If a woman thinks her lover is about to obtain a valuable contract, or a position of authority from the king, or is close to inheriting a fortune, or that his ship will soon arrive laden with merchandise, and if he is always true to his word and keeps his promises . . . then she should have regard for her future welfare and live with him as a wife.

Emergency action

If on the other hand a *Ganika* intends to abandon a particular lover and take up with another one, or when she has reason to believe her lover will shortly leave her and return to his wife, or if her lover is about to lose his job, or, lastly, that he is of very fickle mind . . . then under any of these circumstances she should endeavour to get as much money as she can from him as soon as possible.

On the means of getting money, the signs of change in a lover's feelings, and the way to get rid of him

→>←

M oney is to be got out of a lover in two ways: by lawful means, and by artifices.

Some authorities are of the opinion that when a woman can get as much money as she wants from her lover she should not make use of artifice.

But this author believes that though she may get some money from him by natural means yet when she makes use of artifice he gives her twice as much, and therefore artifice should be employed to extract money from him on all occasions.

Artifices

The artifices to be used for getting money from a lover are as follows:

Taking money from him for the purpose of purchasing such things as ornaments, food, drink, flowers, perfume and clothes and either not buying these, or getting from him more than their cost.
Praising his intelligence to his face.
Pretending to be obliged to make gifts.
Pretending that her jewels have been stolen.
Pretending to have lost the ornaments of her lover along with her own.
Pretending to be ill, and charging the cost of her treatment.
Pretending to sell some of her ornaments or furniture to a trader, who has already been tutored how to behave in this matter.
Lastly, pointing out to her lover the liberality of his rivals.

Warning signs

A woman should always know the feelings of her lover towards her from the changes of his temper, his manner and his face. The behaviour of a waning lover is as follows:

He gives the woman either less than is wanted, or something else.
He pretends to do one thing, and does something else.
He does not fulfil her desires.
He forgets his promises.
He sleeps in some other house under the pretence of having to do something for a friend.
When a woman observes by these actions that her lover's feelings are changing, she should get possession of all his best things before he becomes aware of her intentions, and allow a supposed creditor to take them away forcibly from her in satisfaction of some pretended debt.

Kiss off

The means of getting rid of a lover are as follows:

Describing habits with the sneer of the lip, and the stamp of the foot.
Speaking on a subject with which he is not acquainted.
Seeking the company of men superior to him in learning and wisdom.
Misconstructing his words.
Showing a disregard for him on all occasions.
Interrupting him in the middle of his stories, and beginning other stories herself.
Looking with side glances at her own attendants and clapping her hands when he says anything.
Pretending to be sleepy, not responding to his embraces, keeping her limbs without movement at the time of congress, refusing access to her body.
And, after all these, finally dismissing him.

Conclusion

The duty of a *Ganika* is, after due and full consideration, to form connections with suitable men. After attaching a man to herself she should obtain wealth from him, then dismiss him after she has taken away all his possessions.

PART II
For men – the science of love

+>-<+

The arts of love are dear to women. A man who is skilled in them is looked upon with love by his wife, by the wives of others and by women in society.

A man who employs these arts obtains success and enjoys women of the finest quality.

If broke

A cultivated man who has lost his wealth and has nothing left except his clothes, a razor and some soap should attend parties and social events at the houses of prosperous citizens.

There he will meet women, and if he is skilled in the arts of love he may assure his livelihood without difficulty.

If you can't be rich, be funny

Even if a man is a stranger, unknown, ruined, and without money, if he is liked and trusted he becomes a friend and confidant in rich households and fashionable society.

He will always be welcome if he has the ability to amuse people and make them laugh.

Motive

Apart from pleasure, there are sometimes other reasons for making love to a particular woman. These are:

This woman who loves me has a powerful husband who is a friend of my enemy; she will influence her husband to damage him.

This woman's husband has slept with my wife; I will revenge myself by seducing her.

This woman's rich and powerful husband is hostile; she will turn him in my favour.

This woman is rich and I am poor. To make love to her will enable me to obtain her wealth without difficulty.

After causing this woman to love me we will kill her husband and so obtain his vast riches which I covet.

For these and similar other reasons the wives of other men may sometimes be seduced, but it is wise to avoid the risk merely for the sake of pleasure.

No-nos

The following women are not to be seduced:

A leper.
A lunatic.
A woman who reveals secrets.
A woman who publicly expresses desire for sexual intercourse.
A woman who is extremely white.
A woman who is extremely black.
A woman who smells bad.
A woman who is a close relation.
And, lastly, the wife of a relation, of a friend, of a powerful politician, and the wife of the king.

Size matters

✦✦✦

A man is either a hare, a bull, or a stallion, depending on the size of his *lingam*.

A woman is either a female deer, a mare, or a female elephant, depending on the size and depth of her *yoni*.

In sexual congress the hare with the deer, the bull with the mare, the stallion with the elephant form equal unions. The six other permutations form unequal unions.

Equal unions are the best. The highest with the lowest are the worst. The rest are middling, though the high are better than the low for the male may satisfy his passion without injuring the female, while in the low it is difficult for the female to be satisfied by any means.

Degree of desire . . .
and stamina

≻►⋘

There are also different kinds of union depending upon the force of passion in each partner and the stamina.

When these are similar in the two partners they are well matched; if they are not the pleasure is imperfect.

But here there is a difference of opinion about the female which should be stated. One authority says females do not emit as men do, and this is evident from the fact that males cease after emission and are satisfied, but this is not so with women.

There is however an objection to this opinion, for if a male is long-timed the woman loves him the more, if he be short-timed she is dissatisfied with him. And some say this proves the female emits also.

But this opinion does not hold good, for it takes a long time to allay a woman's desire, and during this time she is enjoying great pleasure. It is therefore quite natural she should wish for its continuation.

Timing and technique

>->-<

On the occasion of first congress the passion of the male is intense and his time short, but in subsequent unions on the same day the reverse is the case. With the female however it is the contrary. The first time her passion is weak and her time long, but on subsequent occasions the same day her passion is intense and her time short until she is satisfied.

Foreplay

--><--

These details particularly apply to married men and their wives. So many men ignore the feelings of women and never pay the slightest attention to their passion. To understand the subject thoroughly it is absolutely necessary to study it, and then a man will know that, as dough is prepared for baking, so must a woman be prepared for sex if she is to derive satisfaction from it.

Reciprocity

On the occasion of first congress kissing, touching and embracing should be done moderately and alternatively. On subsequent occasions, however, moderation is not necessary.

It is believed by some that there is no fixed time or order between the embrace, the kiss and scratching with the nails, but that all these things should be done before sexual congress takes place, while slapping and making the various sounds should occur at the time of union. However, there is another opinion that anything may take place at any time, for love does not care for time or order.

Whatever is done by one of the lovers should be returned by the other. If the woman kisses the man he should kiss her in return, if she slaps him he should also slap her in return.

Scratching and marking

This is not usual except with men and women who are highly passionate, but when love become intense clawing and marking with the nails is practised. This is done on the following occasions:

On the first visit.
At the time of setting out on a journey.
On the return from a journey.
When an angry lover is reconciled.
When the woman is intoxicated.

A caution

A mark of the nails made upon the thighs or breast of a lover is called a 'token of remembrance'.

The marks of nails should not be made on the bodies of married women, but particular kinds of marks may be made on their private parts for the remembrance and increase of love.

Marks of love

The love of a woman who sees the marks of nails on the private parts of her body becomes again fresh and new. If there be no marks to recall the passages of love, then love is lessened, as it is when no union takes place for a long time.

Even when a stranger sees at a distance a young woman with the marks of nails on her breast, he is filled with love and respect for her.

A man also, who carries the marks of nails and teeth on his body, influences the mind of a woman be it ever so firm.

In short, nothing tends to increase love so much as the effects of marking with the nails and biting

*On kissing, scratching,
biting, slapping and the
means to be employed with the
women of different countries*

→>-<←

All parts of the body that can be kissed may also be bitten, except the upper lip, the tongue and the eyes.

As with kissing, scratching etc, those things which increase passion should be done first, and those which are only for amusement or variety should be done afterwards.

Tips for the traveller

In the affairs of love a man should do such things as are agreeable to the women of different countries.

The women of the Balhika country are puritanical but gained over by unusual loveplay. The women of Avantika are fond of foul pleasures and have not good manners. The women of Maharashtra utter low, harsh words, like to be spoken to in the same way, and have an impetuous desire for congress. The women of Malwa are gained over by slapping.

The women of the Punjab are to be won by a particular use of the tongue.

There is an opinion however that the particular pleasure agreeable to a particular woman is of greater importance than the tendency of a whole nation; and it is this which should be followed, rather than the peculiarities of a country.

Reprisal

When a man bites a woman forcibly, she should angrily do the same to him with double force, and if she be excessively chafed she should at once begin a love quarrel with him. She should take hold of her lover by the hair, kiss his lower lip and then, intoxicated by love, bite him in various places.

Even in public, when her lover shows her any mark she may have inflicted on him, she should smile at the sight of it. Then, as if she were going to chide him, she should show him with an angry look the marks on her own body that have been made by him.

Thus, if women and men act to each other's liking, their love for each other will not be lessened even in one hundred years.

Quarrels . . . and reconciliation

→>←←

A woman who is very much in love with a man cannot bear to hear the name of her rival spoken, or to have any conversation regarding her, or to be called by her name through mistake. If this occurs a great quarrel arises. The women becomes angry, tosses her hair about, strikes her lover and, casting aside her ornaments, throws herself down on the ground.

At this time the lover should attempt to reconcile her with conciliatory words, take her up carefully and place her on the bed. But she, not replying to his questions and with increased anger, should pull his hair and, after kicking him thoroughly, should then proceed to the door of the room.

There she should sit and shed tears. After a time, when she thinks the conciliatory words and actions of her lover have reached their utmost, she should then embrace him, reproaching him with harsh words but at the same time showing a loving desire for congress.

Group sex and
diverse practices
→>←←

In Gramaneri it is the custom for many young men to enjoy a woman who may be married to one of them, either one after the other, or at the same time. Thus one of them holds her, another enjoys her, a third uses her mouth, a fourth holds her middle part, and in this way they go on enjoying her in different ways alternately.

The same things can be done when several men are in company with one courtesan, or when one courtesan is alone with many men. In the same way this can be done by the women of the king's harem when they accidentally get hold of a man.

An ingenious person should multiply these diverse practices, for when performed according to the usage of each country and the liking of each individual, they generate love, friendship and respect in the hearts of women.

Mutual abuse

Sexual intercourse can be compared to a quarrel, on account of the contrarieties of love and its tendency to dispute. Slaps and blows given by the man should be returned by the woman, while abusing him as if she were angry.

Because it causes pain, striking gives rise to the hissing sound, and also of words expressing prohibition, sufficiency, desire of liberation, pain or praise.

Women differ from one another greatly. Some like to be talked to in the most loving way, others in the most lustful way, others abusively, and so on. Some enjoy themselves with closed eyes in silence, others make a great noise over it, and some almost faint away.

The great art is to ascertain what gives them the greatest pleasure, and what practices they like best.

Sexual aids

The wedge, the scissors, the piercing instrument, and the pincers may also be employed during sexual congress, but this author is of the opinion that their use is painful, barbarous, base, and quite unworthy of imitation.

Examples of the dangers which result may be given as follows:

The king of the Panchalas killed the courtesan Mádhavasena by means of the wedge during congress; King Satavahana deprived his queen of her life by a pair of scissors; and Naradeva, whose hand was deformed, blinded a dancing girl by directing a piercing instrument in the wrong way.

Role reversal

A woman may act the part of a man when her lover is fatigued, to satisfy his curiosity, or her own desire for novelty.

Though a woman is reserved and keeps her feelings concealed, yet when she acts this way she shows all her love and desire. And a man should gather from her actions of what disposition she is and in what way she likes to be enjoyed herself.

Oral sex

The male servants of some men carry on mouth congress with their masters. It is also practised by some citizens, who know each other well, among themselves.

Some women of the harem, when they are amorous do these acts on one another. And some men do the same thing with women. For the sake of such practices some women will abandon liberal, good, and clever men and become attracted to low persons such as slaves and elephant drivers.

The work of a dog?

Some ancient and venerable authorities hold the opinion that mouth congress is the work of a dog because it is a low practice opposed to the orders of Holy Writ and because the man himself suffers by bringing his *lingam* into contact with the mouths of others.

But this author says the orders of Holy Writ do not affect those who resort to courtesans, and the law prohibits mouth congress only with married women. As regards injury to the male, this can be easily remedied.

A time and a place for everything

Mouth congress should never be performed by a government minister, by a learned Brahman, or a man of good reputation. However there are some occasions where this practice can be made use of. After all, these things are done secretly, and the minds of men and women being fickle, how can it be known what any person may do at any particular time and for any particular purpose?

In conclusion: a man who knows how to do it will be respected and regarded as a leader anywhere

→><←

About those things described there cannot be any fixed rule. Such passionate actions which arise on the spur of the moment during sex cannot be defined and are as irregular as dreams. For this reason one who is well acquainted with the science of love, knowing their own strength and the strength of their partner, should act accordingly.

In conclusion it must be said that though a man may be capable of speaking well on other matters but does not know this science, then little respect will be paid to him in the company of the learned. One who is ignorant of other knowledge but well acquainted with these arts becomes a leader in any group.

Other titles from the 'Illuminations' series

Power
by Machiavelli
The notorious master of the subject sets
out his timeless rules on how to get it, use it
and hold on to it.
ISBN 1 86197 353 5

Happiness
by Marcus Aurelius
The Roman philosopher-emperor describes
his Method to achieve happiness, find inner
peace and change your life for the better.
ISBN 1 86197 367 5

Faith
by St Paul
The renowned spiritual teacher explains
how to find and keep to the path that leads
to life after death.
ISBN 1 86197 372 1